SUBSTANCE ABUSE ASSESSMENT, INTERVENTIONS AND TREATMENT

COCAINE'S IMPACT ON AFFECT, ACTIVITY, AND REWARD IS DOSE-DEPENDENTLY IMPACTED BY AGE

SUBSTANCE ABUSE ASSESSMENT, INTERVENTIONS AND TREATMENT

Additional books in this series can be found on Nova's website under the Series tab.

SUBSTANCE ABUSE ASSESSMENT, INTERVENTIONS AND TREATMENT

COCAINE'S IMPACT ON AFFECT, ACTIVITY, AND REWARD IS DOSE-DEPENDENTLY IMPACTED BY AGE

BRIAN M. KELLEY
CANDACE E. PERRY
HILLARY A. HERSHEY
AND
ADRIANNA L. BAIRD

Nova Science Publishers, Inc.
New York

For permission to use material from this book please contact us:
Telephone 631-231-7269; Fax 631-231-8175
Web Site: http://www.novapublishers.com

NOTICE TO THE READER

Additional color graphics may be available in the e-book version of this book.

Library of Congress Cataloging-in-Publication Data

Cocaine's impact on affect, activity, and reward are dose-dependently impacted by age / editors, Brian M. Kelley ... [et al.].
p. cm.
Includes index.
ISBN 978-1-61122-744-4 (hardcover)
1. Cocaine. 2. Cocaine abuse--Age factors. I. Kelley, Brian M.
QP801.C68C666 2010
362.29'8--dc22
2010041354

Published by Nova Science Publishers, Inc. † New York

Contents

Preface

The purpose of the present study is to examine the impact of different doses of cocaine on three interrelated measures related to affective behaviors between adolescent and adult mice. In order to assess the range of affective and rewarding responses, measure of despair, activity, and reward were used. Such methods included the forced swim test (FST), motor activity (MA), and the conditioned place preference (CPP) tests, respectively. Cocaine was selected, in part, because of its robust psychostimulant properties, its use by millions of substance abusers worldwide, and its well understood mechanism of action. The results show that adolescents have an increased sensitivity to cocaine's ability to alleviate despair compared to adults in the forced swim test. The adolescents showed a decreased sensitivity to the drug in the motor activity and conditioned place preference tests. The clinical implications of this study support an enormous body of clinical research, which suggest that substance abuse is primarily initiated during adolescence and that it often co-occurs with affective disorders. This study may help explain some of the neurobiological underpinnings of these finding because cocaine was especially effective in reducing despair-related behavior in adolescence compared with adults, yet less effective as an euphoric agent. This is the worst possible finding because it suggests that adolescents will find cocaine particularly effective in alleviating negative mood states resulting in increased use; however, in order to achieve euphoria higher doses will be required. The combination of these effects place youth at a particular disadvantage compared with adults and, as such, places them at a greater risk for lifelong substance abuse problems.

Chapter I

Introduction

Drug experimentation, which is almost universally initiated during adolescents, often results in a plethora of primary and secondary adverse events impacting the substance user, their family, and their community as well as involving local, state, and federal agencies. While the personal costs associated to substance abuse problems are immeasurable, recent estimates suggest that substance abuse related problems cost the United States over $484 billion per year (Anderson, 2005). The nearly half a trillion dollars spent per year includes only health care expenditures, lost earnings, and costs associated with crime and accidents and does not reflect the high economic burden substance abuse places on the family (e.g., divorce, child abuse, parental absence, reduced academic support, etc.; Anderson 2005). Drug abuse related cost greatly exceeds those associated with chronic conditions such as cancer and diabetes for which the United States spends a comparatively small $171.6 billion and $131.7 billion, respectively (Anderson, 2005).

Given that substance abuse is such a widespread problem, the U.S. Government invests approximately $1.5 billion on prevention programs per year with no foreseeable reduction in sight (Carelzon, Mague, and Anderson, 2003). While prevention efforts are costly, they nearly always produce a positive impact as current studies show a reduction in use across most categories of abused drugs, with the principle exceptions including inhalants and prescription drugs. According to Substance Abuse and Mental Health Services Administration's (SAMHSA) National Survey on Drug Use and Health (2008), among youths aged 12 to 17, the types of drugs used in the past month varied by age group with 1.5 percent of 12 to 13 years olds using prescription-type drugs for non medical purposes, 1.2 percent using inhalants, and 1.0 percent used marijuana. Slightly older adolescents, those age 14 to 15 years, most commonly used marijuana (5.7 %), followed by nonmedical use of prescription-type drugs (3.0 %), inhalants (1.3 %), and hallucinogens (1.0 %). Marijuana also was the most commonly used drug among 16 or 17 year olds (12.7 %); it was followed by nonmedical use of prescription-type drugs (4.0 %), hallucinogens (1.6 %), cocaine (0.7 %), and inhalants (0.7 %).

With respect to alcohol, a little more than half of Americans aged 12 and older reported being current drinkers, more than one fifth (23.3 percent) participated in binge drinking at least once in the 30 days prior to the survey, and heavy drinking was reported by 6.9 percent of the population sampled. Lastly, in this same survey, an estimated 70.9 million Americans aged 12 and older were current (past month) tobacco users. This represents 28.4 percent of the population in this age range. In addition, 59.8 million persons (23.9 percent of the population) were current cigarette smokers; 13.1 million (5.3 percent) smoked cigars; 8.7 million (3.5 percent) used smokeless tobacco; and 1.9 million (0.8 percent) smoked tobacco in pipes. The average age for first use of an abused substance was about 15 years for inhalants, 16 years for alcohol, 17 years for nicotine, and about 19 years for illicit drugs. The pattern of use noted in this survey and other similar studies (Kandel et al., 1992) offer direct evidence that substance abuse is a pediatric disease. Furthermore, such evidence provides convincing evidence of the "gateway model of drug abuse," which suggests the typical pattern of substance use is to start with more conventional, legal, and readily available substances (e.g., nicotine, alcohol, and inhalants) followed by a systematic elevation in the type of drug abused, like illicit drugs (e.g., marijuana, cocaine, methamphetamine, heroin, and ecstasy).

This phenomenon, termed the "gateway drug effect," has been well documented (O'Donnell, 1979; Johnston, 1986; Johnston et al., 1987; Kandel et al., 1992; Torabi et al., 1993). One study noted a dose-dependent relationship between smoking and binge drinking and illicit drug use. In particular, daily, pack-a-day smokers were three times more likely to drink alcohol, seven times more likely to use smokeless tobacco, and ten to thirty times more likely to use illicit drugs compared to non-smokers (Torabi et al., 1993).

The culmination of these and similar findings have serious implications considering initiating substance use during adolescence is correlated with an increase in severity of dependence, greater addiction liability, higher daily consumption, and reduced probability of quitting (Taioli and Wynder, 1991; Breslua and Peterson, 1996; Chen and Millar, 1998; Spear, 2000; Chambers et al., 2003). Also, escalation of drug use is more rapid and the risk of dependence is greater in adolescents than adults as well (Estroff et al., 1989; Robins and Przybeck, 1995; Chen et al., 1997; Clark et al.,1998). The escalation from tobacco, inhalants, alcohol, or prescription drugs use to illicit drug use, abuse and dependence may include factors beyond the obvious sociocultural factors (e.g., peer pressure, advertising, media, etc.). It is possible, even probable, that the "gateway" effect may be due, in part, to neurochemical alterations in reward systems. Hence, adolescent substance use could serve as a neurochemical "gateway" for subsequent drug abuse and dependence.

The elevation in substance use, abuse, and dependence noted during adolescents has increasingly been shown to be associated with rather remarkable changes in brain processes. For example, across adolescent development the central nervous system is subject to dramatic changes in hormone levels, synaptic pruning, apoptosis, cell replication and migration, as well as the functional programming of behavioral responses (Altman and Bayer 1990; Bayer, Yackel, and Puri 1982; Huttenlocher 1990; McWilliams and Lynch 1983; Rezvani and Levin 2004; Scheetz 1994; Spear and Brake 1983). Similarly, changes in brain processes are associated with a unique pattern of behavior including increased rates of novelty seeking, risk taking, exploration, impulsivity, social behavior, and aggression (Spear, 2000). Markedly, these processes are impacted by a broad spectrum of pharmacological agents that can disrupt and impair development (Slotkin 2004; Spear 2000). To this end and in support of the "neurochemical gateway effect", previous research in our laboratory has shown that adolescent nicotine exposure permanently alters reward systems of adult mice thus placing nicotine-exposed subjects at greater risk for drug abuse problems throughout life (Kelley and Middaugh, 1999; Kelley and Rowan, 2004; Nolley, and Kelley, 2007). So, contrary to the customary observation that adolescence is part of a continuum of change (i.e., from childhood to adulthood), evidence now suggests that adolescence is instead a unique developmental period, which is particularly vulnerable to substance use initiation and drug insults.

The rapid neurobiological changes that transpire during adolescence not only elevate risk for substance abuse problems, such changes also increase the risk for and incidence of affective disorders. As a matter of fact, adolescence is the period of highest risk for the onset of depression (Burke et al., 1990). At any given time, 5–8% of adolescents meet the criteria for major depressive disorder (Lewinsohn et al., 1994). Specifically, elevated risk for depression begins in the early teens and continues to rise in a linear fashion throughout adolescence. More specifically, population-based studies show the prevalence rate to be between 0.4 to 2.5 percent for children (under 12), 0.7 to 9.8 percent during early adolescence, and between 15-25 percent during late adolescence (Ciaconia et al., 1994; Hankin et al., 1998; Weissman, et al., 1995). Unfortunately, too many adolescents deal with negative affective states by using a variety of readily available substances, which may offer immediate, short-term relief for such states. The self-medication hypothesis of substance abuse, also known as comorbidity or dual diagnosis, suggests that a person abuses particular drugs because of their potential to reduce negative emotional states, improve cognitive performance, or manage psychological problems.

This hypothesis predicts that users seek out specific drugs, which make them feel "normal," to use and then abuse (Woodward and Fergusson, 2001; Rounsaville, 2004). According to contemporary research, 30 to 60 percent of drug abusers have coexisting psychological problems. Large-scale research suggests that the most common disorders diagnosed along with drug dependence are personality disorders, anxiety disorders, and depression (Compton, Cottler, Jacobs, Ben-Abdalian, and Spitznagel, 2003).

In this scenario, difficulties multiple because the consequences of substance use and abuse often create or exacerbate psychological problems, which can occur during the drug and/or withdrawal state (Makkai, 2003).

Considering the rapid availability and wide variety of drugs accessible to our youth, it is not surprising to find substance use and abuse associated with exogenous attempts to modify or control negative affective states, especially considering such states may be comparatively new experiences for teens (i.e., at least in terms of intensity and frequency). The neuroanatomical and neurochemical substrates involved in substance abuse and affective disorders have tremendous overlap (e.g., amygdala, prefrontal cortex, hippocampus, and nucleus accumbens as well as dopamine, norepinephrine, and serotonin, respectively) and all show tremendous development and refinement during adolescence.

While the neurodevelopmental processes that contribute to the physiological, behavioral, cognitive, and affective differences between adolescents and adults are not well understood, some studies suggest these differences to be principally mediated by a differential degree of maturation of dopaminergic systems in the brain, especially within the limbic system (Shalaby et al, 1981; Spear and Brake, 1983; Kalsbeek et al, 1988; Teicher et al, 1995).

In support of this hypothesis it has been shown that dopamine content, fiber density, and dopamine receptors reach peak levels during adolescence and undergo pruning in several brain regions thereafter (Hohn and Wuttke, 1979; Kalsbeek et al, 1988; Lidow et al, 1991; Teicher et al, 1995; Tarazi et al, 1999). In the present study, we have chosen to focus on cocaine's effects on the dopaminergic system to allow for a more comprehensive investigation of its effect on reward mechanisms in adolescent and adult mice. Because cocaine influences dopaminergic systems, because dopaminergic systems are important for the reinforcing effects of nearly all abused drugs, because dopaminergic systems are rapidly developing during adolescence, and because developing systems are particularly sensitive to insult (Vorhees, 1994), it is probable that adolescents may differ from adults across behaviors mediated by dopaminergic systems and these system may be especially sensitive to insult.

An ever growing body of literature is mounting noting the differential sensitivity to cocaine in adolescent and adult rodents (Laviola et al, 1995; Philpot and Kirstein, 1999; Collins and Izenwasser, 2002; Ehrlich et al, 2002; Stansfield and Kirstein, 2005; Frantz et al, 2007). For instance, adolescent rats given an acute challenge with cocaine demonstrate a larger dopaminergic response in the nucleus accumbens compared with adult rats and do so in a manner that is contingent upon the degree of novel object exploration, a tentative measure of impulsivity (Stansfield and Kirstein, 2005).

Repeated cocaine exposure has been reported to produce a leftward shift in dopamine responsiveness in nucleus accumbens of adolescent rats as compared to acute cocaine administration (Philpot and Kirstein, 1999; Badanich et al, 2006). However, with regards to the effects of repeated cocaine exposure, not all studies have produced similar results. For example, Frantz et al (2007) compared the motor and reinforcing effects of cocaine in adolescents and adults Wistar rats and measured extracellular dopamine in the nucleus accumbens of both groups following a cocaine challenge.

Although these investigators found age-related differences in behavioral activity, no differences were observed in increases in extracellular dopamine levels in the nucleus accumbens produced by cocaine. On the other hand, Cao et al. (2007) showed that adolescent rats were less sensitive to the ability of cocaine to elevate extracellular levels of dopamine in the nucleus accumbens as compared with adults.

The rationale for testing cocaine in adolescent and adult mice across a number of important and related behaviors is twofold. First, in 2008, 5.3 million Americans age 12 and older had abused cocaine in some form and 1.1 million had abused crack at least once in the year prior to being surveyed (SAMSHA, 2008). Similarly, the 2008 Monitoring the Future Study showed that 1.8 percent of 8th graders, 3.0 percent of 10th graders, and 4.4 percent of 12th graders had abused cocaine in some form and 1.1 percent of 8th graders, 1.3 percent of 10th graders, and 1.6 percent of 12th graders had abused crack at least once in the year prior to being surveyed (Monitoring the Future, 2008). From an epidemiological standpoint, the powerful psychostimulant properties of cocaine are known to impact a great many users and such use is associated with a range of violent and premature deaths. Second, cocaine's mechanism of action is associated with tremendous elevations in dopamine, norepinephrine, and serotonin levels in brain regions thought to be important for all abused drugs (Wise and Bozarth, 1987; Koob, 1992; Di Chiara, 1995) and affective disorders and, as such, can serve as a prototypical agent by which other drugs can be compared.

While studies have addressed both the questions of inherent differences between adolescence and adulthood and the extended consequences of adolescent drug exposures, it remains unclear if adolescent compared with adult mice show dissimilar patterns of behavior across important measures of affect, activity, and reward. Thus, the purpose of the present study was to examine differences in response to a cocaine dose-response curve in adolescent and adult mice using the forced swim test, measures of locomotor activity, and conditioned place preference.

The use of several interrelated measures, in the same subjects, will provide converging validation of behaviors known to be important for dopaminergic function. Lastly, this study is the first to provide measures across a continuum of affective states from despair to motor activation to reward in the same subjects, including adolescent and adult subjects, in response to a cocaine dose-response curve.

Chapter II

Methods

Drug Source and Administration

Saline and cocaine were purchased from Sigma Chemical Company, St. Louis, MO. All drugs were administered at an injection volume of 0.01 ml/g body weight. Prepared in physiological saline, cocaine was administered by means of intraperitoneal injection. Cocaine dissolved in physiological saline was administered intraperitoneally 10 minutes prior to testing. This time was selected based on known rate of cocaine absorption and metabolism. For each experiment, control groups received vehicle injections, with testing following identical time parameters.

Subjects

This experiment was completed in accordance with the guidelines enforced by the Guide for the Care and Use of Laboratory Animals, set by the National Institutes of Health. For this experiment, a total of 96 male C57BL/6J (C57; Jackson Laboratory, Bar Harbor, Maine) were used. Of this sample, 48 were adolescents that arrived on postnatal day 21, and 48 were adults that arrived on postnatal day 85.

We defined periadolescence as inclusive of the period occurring immediately before, during, and immediately after puberty. Periadolescence in rodents has not been clearly defined in any research study, but the most commonly used time frame is postnatal day 21 to postnatal day 50. Our study began testing on postnatal day 25, with the last test performed on postnatal day 50, assuring that all of our non-adult subjects were within the periadolescent time frame. A rodent enters adulthood between postnatal days 65-75. To ensure that adult subjects were in fact adults, testing began on postnatal day 89.

All subjects were individually housed upon delivery, and were maintained in a temperature controlled environment 22 C with a 12 h light-dark cycle (lights from 7 PM to 7 AM) and allowed free access to food and water. Following a four-day acclimation period, subjects were assigned to one of four treatment groups. For four days, beginning with postnatal day 25 for adolescents and postnatal day 89 for adults, subjects received intraperitoneal injections of saline or 5.0, 10.0, 20.0, or 40.0 mg/kg cocaine, according to the design of each method.

Forced Swim Test

The forced swim test consisted of six minute sessions over a period four days. Each subject was placed into a standard 1500 ml swim chamber filled with 1200 ml of clean, room temperature water. Swim chambers, located in an adjacent room, were placed under a ventilation hood that served to eliminate the scent of other subjects being tested and any additional odors. It also provided white masking noise. All sessions were videotaped for subsequent data analysis and were timed using a stopwatch. The forced swim test (FST) is a widely accepted animal model used to screen drugs for antidepressant activity (Porsolt et al., 1977). Although different classes of antidepressants produce diverse neurochemical and neurobiological effects, the FST is a good predictor of the clinical efficacy of antidepressants or drugs known to elevate mood (Willner, 1990; Detke et al., 1995; Cryan et al., 2002).

Motor Activity Apparatus

The motor activity monitoring system was located in a testing room adjacent to the colony room and each of the four monitoring systems was placed in a sound attenuation chamber that included a white noise generator and a 20W light. Motor activity was measured with a Digiscan Animal Activity Monitoring System (Model RXYZCM8 TAO, Coulbourn Instruments) with a two animal option. The apparatus consisted of eight 20 cm × 20 cm Plexiglas chambers (i.e., two per monitor). Activity was measured by interruption of infrared photo beams. Programming allows for quantification of locomotion (distance traveled in cm) as well as other variables. While this system can quantify numerous outcome measures, these measure (e.g., rest time, movement time, and stereotypy) tend to be highly correlated, either positively or negatively with one another, and the scientific value of some of these measures remains to be validated (i.e., stereotypy). We selected the most objective measure, cm traveled, for this study. Data, which is processed by the Digiscan Analyzer and fed via an interface system into a computer, was collected in 5 min intervals across the 30 min test sessions.

Conditioned-Place-Preference Apparatus

Conditioned-place-preference testing apparatus consisted of four Plexiglas chambers (46 cm x 24 cm x 22 cm) and was located in a testing room adjacent to the colony room. A removable partition divided each chamber into two equal sized distinguishable compartments; one black and the other white. Subjects were acclimated to the apparatus for one day, prior to actual testing, with no partition for twenty minutes. There was a total of ten sessions, where data was collected. The first day served as the pre-test, where subjects were placed in the chamber with an open partition, so they could freely explore the chamber. Preference was recorded to total number of seconds each subject in either the black or white side of the chamber. The subject was considered to have entered a side once three paws had crossed the midline. Then, over a period of eight days, each subject was administered saline when placed in their recorded preferred side, and administered cocaine when placed in their recorded non-preferred side. Each session lasted for a total of twenty minutes, with a closed partition. Following this eight-day period, a single post-test was performed, in which subjects were placed in the chamber with an open partition, similar to the procedure utilized in the pre-test. The post-test was performed to see if the previous eight days had had an effect on each subject's preferred side. The post-test was to indicate if the pairing of cocaine had produced a change in preference.

Experiment

Experiment one: forced swim test. After the four-day acclimation period, subjects were placed on an AABA design, receiving saline on the first and second days of the design, cocaine on the third day, and then saline again on the fourth day. After completion of all four days, data was analyzed according to time spent climbing, swimming, and immobility. Three researchers reviewed the videotapes of the subjects, each using a stopwatch to determine how much time was spent performing each behavior. Albeit considerably more time-intensive, this method of quantifying forced-swim test behavior is much more accurate than conventional methods. In previous reports, researchers observed the subjects in five-minute increments and simply categorized each 5 second period based on the most predominant behavior. While this method is efficient in behavioral screening procedures for assessing the putative antidepressant effect of novel chemicals, the potential exists to lose up half of the data (e.g., if a subject is observed swimming for 2.4 seconds but climbing for 2.6 seconds, then the entire 5-second increment is scored as climbing).

For the purposes of this study, three experienced technicians watched the video recording of the FST and recorded how much time a subject was engaged in one of the three behaviors; that is, each technician recorded only one behavior. During recording, each technician was blind to the treatment condition and the other technician's data until completion of the recording. Measurements that were off by more than 5 seconds for the entire trial were repeated. Because the behaviors are relatively easy to define and observe, coding of the data was uneventful.

Despite minor differences in scoring, other aspects of the procedure were identical to previous reports. Consistent with previous studies, climbing was defined as vertical movement of the subject, where both forepaws are in contact with the swim chamber. Swimming was defined as movement throughout the swim chamber, crossing quadrants, or using movements that were necessary to keep the subject's head above water. Immobility was defined as movements that served only as a means of keeping the subject's head above water, lasting for at least two seconds. These observational definitions were derived from the methods of Cryan, Valentino, and Lucki (Chambers, Taylor, and Potenza, 2003). Mice were divided across 4 test conditions in accordance with the 4 doses of cocaine tested; thus, forced swim testing was a between subject design. Again, it is important to note that the way in which the forced swim test was conducted for this particular study is somewhat different compared with previous studies.

Whereas this study's method was much more labor intensive, others are more efficient but could lead to a potential loss of up to 49% of all data. The method used in this study ensured a very minimal amount of data could be lost by potential rounding errors, with only a 5-second margin of error. At the same time, however, this intense method of measuring the three FST behaviors (i.e., swimming, climbing, and immobility) made the overall study more complex, requiring more time and effort in order to guarantee a more accurate and complete presentation of data. Subsequent studies interested in sensitivity differences across the FST, compared with more conventional antidepressant screening methods, may be interested in adopting the methodology noted in this study.

Experiment two: motor activity. This portion of the experiment began with an acclimation day, in which subjects were injected with saline, and placed in the motor activity apparatus for 30 minutes, with no data collection. Over the next ten days, data was collected. Saline was administered to all subjects for the first three days of data collection. On the fourth, sixth, eighth, and tenth day, all subjects received the same increasing doses of cocaine (5.0, 10.0, 20.0, and 40.0 mg/kg respectively) and were placed in the motor activity apparatus for a total of 30 minutes of data. Subjects were administered saline on the fifth, seventh, and ninth day as control conditions. While the monitoring system is capable of detecting numerous movements, most are highly correlated, while some are subject to controversy based upon minor differences in operational definitions. For these reasons, cm traveled was used as the principle measure as it represents the most objective measure of locomotor activity. All subjects received each dose of cocaine across the schedule noted above; thus, locomotor activity testing was carried out by way of a repeated measures, within subjects design.

Experiment three: conditioned-place preference. Testing was first initiated with a one-day acclimation trial. Thereafter, a pre-test day followed, which was used to determine initial side preferences. This was followed by eight days of alternating cocaine and saline administration, which was counter-balanced across age and dose. This testing period ended with a post-test day, as previously described. Mice were divided across 4 test conditions in accordance with the 4 doses of cocaine tested; thus, conditioned-place-preference testing was by way of a between subject design. Overall Design: Subjects were randomly assigned to one of four cocaine dose conditions. Subjects tested with the 5.0 dose of cocaine for the forced swim test received the same dose for conditioned-place-preference testing. This was also the case for subjects tested at the other three cocaine doses (10, 20, and 40 mg/kg). However, all mice, irrespective of dose condition for the forced swim and conditioned-place-preference tests, received each of the four doses of cocaine for locomotor activity tests in the pattern noted above. By the nature of the forced swim and condition-place-preference tests (i.e., testing on one day would dramatically impact all subsequent testing), they had to be carried out in a between subjects design; however, this is not the case with locomotor activity testing (e.g., within subject design).

Chapter III

Results

Forced Swim Test: Saline Control Days: Climbing, Immobility, and Swimming

Because each mouse followed the same pattern of saline testing across the four days of forced swim testing, their saline days were collapsed across dose condition as to provide more power. Data is presented as raw data and noted in Figure 1. An ANOVA comparing the saline control days in the FST for the variable Climbing (upper panel) was carried out and the results noted a significant difference across days [$F(2, 180) = 22.89$, $p = 0.0001$] as well as an interaction of days x age [$F(2, 180) = 9.54$, $p = 0.0001$].

A post-hoc analysis, using the Fisher LSD test, of days noted significant difference between the adolescent and adult subjects at day 1 and day 2 but not at day 3; also, adolescent mice showed no difference between days 1 and 2 but did from day 2 to 3, while the opposite pattern was noted in adults.

The variable Immobility (middle panel) showed a significant main effect for Days [$F(2, 178) = 39.28$, $p = 0.0001$] as well as a significant interaction of Days x Age [$F(2, 180) = 4.93$, $p = 0.008$].

Adolescent subjects showed reduced Immobility compared to Adult subjects across the Day 1 and Day 2 but not Day 3 as revealed by Fisher LSD post-hoc analysis. Also, post-hoc tests showed significant increases in Immobility, for adolescent subjects, from day 1 to Day 2 and from Day 2 to Day 3, while adults showed an increase only from Day 1 to Day 2.

An ANOVA comparing the saline control days in the FST for the variable Swimming (bottom panel) noted a significant main effect for days [$F(2 ,180) = 20.84$, $p = 0.0001$] with the adolescent subject's showing higher levels of swimming compared to adults; however, there was no significant interaction of Days x Age. Post-hoc analysis, using the Fisher LSD test, demonstrated that the adolescent subjects continued to show a drop in Swimming from Day 1 to Day 2 and from Day 2 to Day 3, while the adults only showed a significant change in Swimming from Day 1 to Day 2.

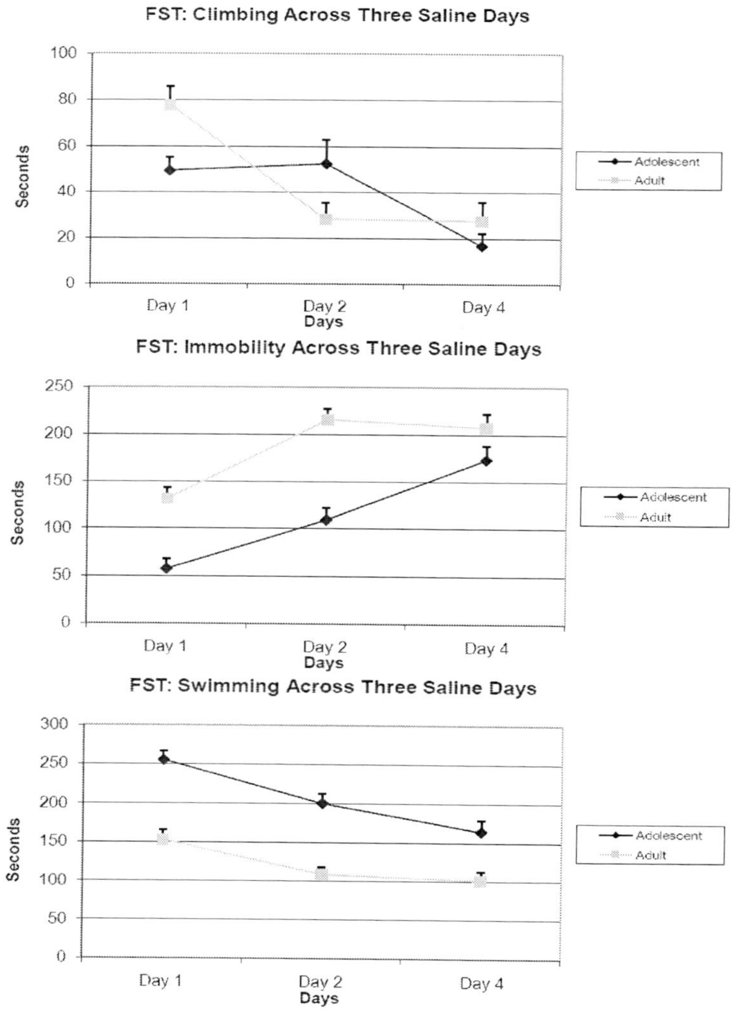

Figure 1. The effects of saline (IP injection) on climbing, immobility, and swimming in the forced swim test (within subjects design). Data is graphed in seconds engaged in climbing, immobility, and swimming (mean ± S.E.).

Dose Response Curve: Climbing, Immobility, and Swimming

Data for the FST cocaine dose-response curve is presented as raw data in Figure 2. There was a significant main effect for Age [$F(1, 83) = 4.20$, $p = 0.04$] in the analysis of Climbing (upper panel) as noted by ANOVA. Further, the interaction of Age x Dose was also significant [$F(3, 91) = 3.15$, $p = 0.029$]. The main effect Dose was not significant. Post-hoc tests showed that the adolescent subjects Climbed significantly more at the 5.0 and 20.0 mg/kg doses of cocaine compared to adults. Difference data equaled the cocaine dose minus the previous saline control day. Analysis of the difference data (Figure 3) for the variable Climbing (upper panel) revealed a significant main effect for Age [$F(1, 83) = 34.316$, $p = 0.0001$] and Dose[$F(3, 83) = 2.856$, $p = 0.04$] as well as a significant interaction of Age x Dose[$F(3, 91) = 3.37$, $p = 0.02$]. Post-hoc tests showed that the adults climbed less than the adolescents at every dose of cocaine but 10.0 mg/kg. Also, the adults did not show a significant change in Climbing across dose; however, the adolescent subject's showed a reduction in climbing from the 5.0 to the 10.0 mg/kg dose and an increase from the 10.0 to the 20.0 mg/kg dose of cocaine.

Immobility (Figure 2, middle panel) was impacted by Age [$F(1, 83) = 54.384$, $p = 0.0001$] and Dose [$F(3, 83) = 4.467$, $p = 0.006$] and the interaction of Age x Dose approached significance [$F(3, 91) = 2.478$, $p = 0.067$], as revealed by ANOVA. Post-hoc analysis showed that the adolescent subjects engaged in less Immobility compared to adults at every dose but the lowest and even at this dose the difference approached significance (0.07).

The adult subjects showed no significant change in Immobility across dose; however, the adolescent subjects showed a reduction across the dose-response curve, most notably at the two highest doses of cocaine (20.0 and 40.0 mg/kg compared to the lowest two doses, 5.0 and 10.0 mg/kg respectively).

These findings were further magnified by the analysis of the difference values (Figure 3, middle panel). Both Age [$F(1, 83) = 2.72$, $p = 0.05$] and Dose [$F(3, 83) = 8.47$, $p = 0.005$] as well as the interaction of Age x Dose [$F(3, 91) = 2.78$, $p = 0.48$] were significant. Post-hoc tests showed that, compared to adults, adolescents showed less immobility at the 10.0 and 20.0 mg/kg doses of cocaine. Also, the general finding for adolescents was a reduction in immobility, whereas, for adults, there was either no effect or an increase, as noted at the 10.0 mg/kg dose of cocaine.

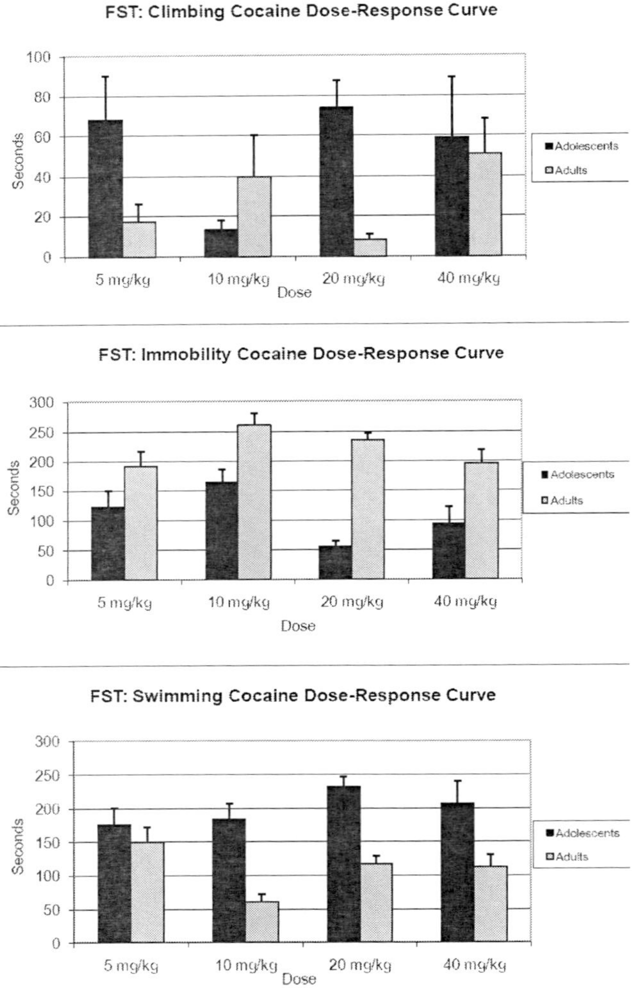

Figure 2. The effects of acute cocaine (5.0, 10.0, 20.0, and 40 mg/kg, IP injection) on climbing, immobility, and swimming in the forced swim test (between subjects design). Data is graphed in seconds engaged in climbing, immobility, and swimming (mean ± S.E.).

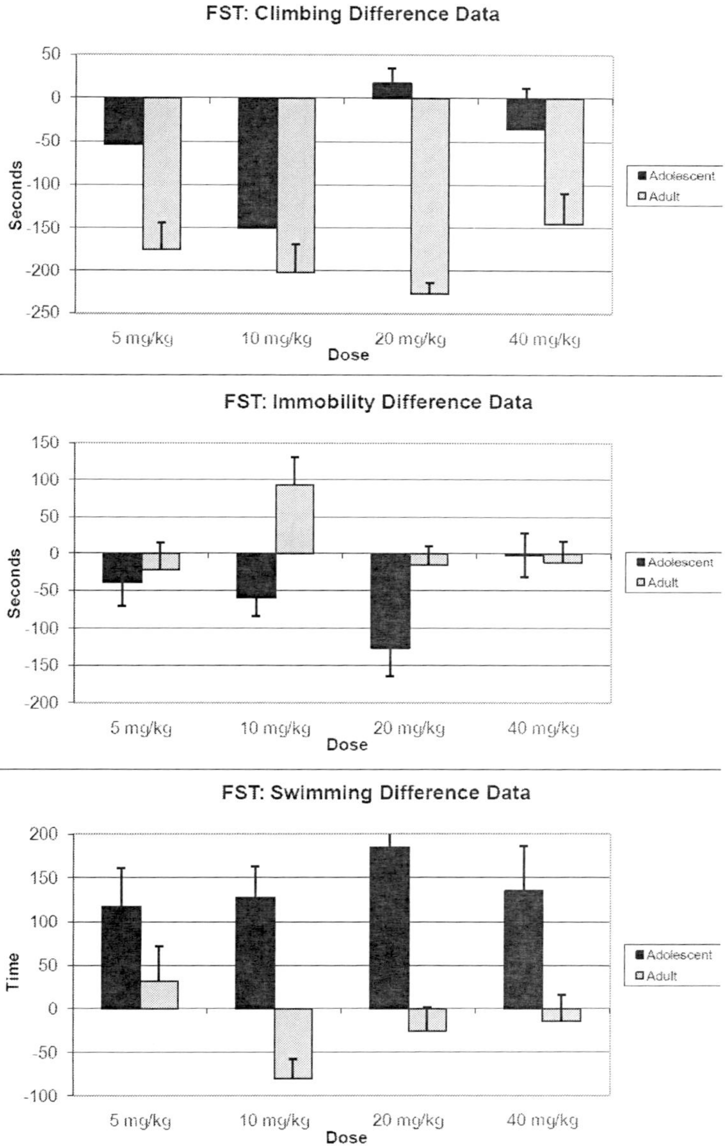

Figure 3. The effects of acute cocaine (5.0, 10.0, 20.0, and 40 mg/kg, IP injection) on climbing, immobility, and swimming in the forced swim test (between subjects design). Data is graphed as the seconds difference between the cocaine dose-previous saline control data for climbing, immobility, and swimming (mean ± S.E.).

A significant main effect for Age [F(1, 83) = 37.69, p = 0.0001] was noted from ANOVA for the raw data across the cocaine dose-response curve for the variable Swimming (Figure 2, bottom panel). The main effect for Dose [F(3, 83) = 37.69, p = 0.0.073] approached significance as did the interaction of Age x Dose [F(3,91) = 2.247, p = 0.089. Post-hoc tests, using the Fisher LSD, showed that the adolescent subjects Swam significantly more compared to adults across all but the lowest dose of cocaine. Analysis of the difference data (Figure 3, bottom panel), showed a main effect for Age [F(1, 83) = 46.28, p = 0.0001], no other analysis were significant. Post-hoc tests, again using the Fisher LSD, noted that the Adolescent subjects Swam significantly more than the adults at every dose but the lowest.

Motor Activity

Motor activity data is presented as raw data in Figure 4. Motor activity data was analyzed using a mixed between, within repeated measures ANOVA; specifically, a 2 (Age: Adolescent vs. Adult) x 5 (Dose: Cocaine 0, 5, 10, 20, and 40 mg/kg) x 6 (Time: 5, 10, 15, 20, 25, and 30 minutes) with Age as the between factor and Dose and Time as repeated factors.

The ANOVA showed a significant main effect for Dose [F(4, 344) = 48.528, p = 0.0001) and Time [F(5,430) = 171.29, p = 0.0001] and significant interactions for Time x Age [,F(5,430) = 4.31, p= 0.0001] and Dose x Time [F(20,1720) = 6.83, p= 0.0001]. The full interaction approached significance [F(20,1720) = 1.42, p = 0.10]. Fishers LSD post-hoc tests showed that Adolescent subjects had a more rapid drop in activity across increasing time compared to adults. This was noted most prominently at lower and higher doses. Further, an analysis of slope at each dose showed a significant effect ($p < 0.05$) with Adolescent subjects showing a steeper slope at each dose compared with Adults.

Conditioned Place Preference

A 2 (Age: Adolescent vs Adult) x 4 (Cocaine Dose: 5, 10, 20, and 40 mg/kg) ANOVA revealed a significant main effect for Age [F(1,78) = 7.349 p = 0.008]. Post-hoc analysis with Fishers LSD test showed a reduction in conditioning at the 10.0 and the 20.0 mg/kg doses compared to Adults. Differences between Adolescents and Adults was further supported by an analysis of slope (p = 0.0001), with Adults showing an overall positive slope compared with Adolescents showing the opposite pattern.

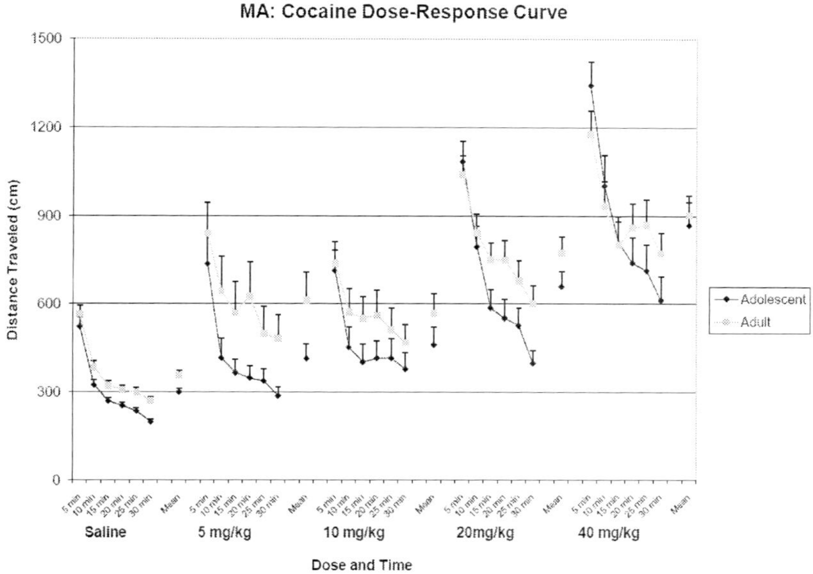

Figure 4. The effects of acute cocaine (5.0, 10.0, 20.0, and 40 mg/kg, IP injection) on motor activity of adolescent and adult subjects (within subjects design). Data is graphed as cm traveled (mean ± S.E.).

Chapter IV

Conclusion

Our general findings note innate differences between adolescent and adult mice across measures of affective states and motor activity. Related to cocaine exposure, our findings note an interaction between cocaine sensitivity and age across a dose-response curve and across a continuum from negative to positive affect with adolescent, compared to adults, showing an increased response to alleviating despair and a decreased response to reward. Furthermore, both measures of affect included a learned element, both operant and classical conditioning, in contrast to motor activity, which is an unconditioned measure of cocaine sensitivity. The unlearned responses noted during motor activity testing show a tendency for adolescent subjects' to show a less robust psychostimulant effect and, more specifically, for motor activity levels to drop off more rapidly within and across different cocaine doses compared with adults. In summary, the data suggests neurobiological difference across developmental account for altered responses to cocaine in adolescent subjects compared to adults subjects.

Chapter V

Discussion

Overall findings include the diminished sensitivity of adolescents to despair in the FST. In contrast, a greater response in alleviation of despair was seen with cocaine in adolescents when compared to adults. Across the saline days, significant differences were found between adolescents and adults. As can be seen in the FST: Control Day Values, Immobility Graph, a difference can be seen on day 1 with the adolescent subjects spending significantly less time immobile than adults. By day 2, adolescent subjects demonstrate an even greater difference in immobility than adult subjects; however, both groups experience a significant increase in time spent across this measure. The adults show a 64 percent increase, while the adolescents show an 88 percent increase. At day 4 (the day after cocaine was administered), no difference is seen between the two groups. The adults show a non-significant drop in time spent immobile (a mere 3 percent difference), while the adolescents continue to show a significant increase, spending 59 percent more time immobile than on the second saline day. The adolescents show an overall 200 percent increase in immobility across the saline days, while the adults showed only a 58 percent increase. The differences in immobility cannot be accounted for by innate differences in activity as adolescent mice showed lower levels of baseline activity in motor testing, albeit the difference was modest compared with adults. One interpretation is that adolescent mice are more resilient in this particular task. However, it is possible that the increase in time for both groups could have been a learned/adaptive response. That is, if the FST is a measure of learned helplessness, it is possible to interpret the data as faster learning in adults suggesting that adolescent subjects are less capable of adapting to repeated stress.

Whereas the adults spent more time immobile, the adolescents spent more time swimming. This was expected; if the adolescents spent less time being immobile than the adults, they had to have spent more time engaging in one of the other two behaviors (e.g., swimming or climbing). As seen in the FST: Control Day Values, Swimming Graph, at day 2, the adolescents show a significant decrease in time spent swimming with a 21 percent difference from day 1. The adults also show a significant decrease in swim time, with a 28 percent difference. At day 4, the adolescents show another significant decrease, spending 17 percent less time swimming. The adults also show a decrease, however, it was not statistically significant. This overall decreasing pattern seen in Swimming Graph for both groups corresponds with the overall increasing pattern seen in immobility. For swimming across all saline days, the adolescents show an overall 35 percent decrease, while the adults shown a 33 percent decrease; so, while the adolescents clearly swim less, they show a similar pattern of activity, compared with adults, across the three control days.

As can be seen in FST: Control Day Values, Climbing Graph, both groups spent less time climbing than swimming. That said, some significant differences were still noted. On day 1, the adults spent significantly more time in the climbing phase. On day 2, a significant difference is still seen between the two groups. The adults show a significant decrease, spending 63%less time than the day before. A slight increase is seen with the adolescents; however, it is not significant. At day 4, the difference seen between the two groups is not significant. The adults again show a decrease in climbing, but it is not significant with only a 2% difference. The adolescents, on the other hand, show a significant decrease, spending 67% less time climbing than on the 2nd day. From day 1 to day 4, the adolescents show an overall 65% decrease in time spent climbing, while the adults show a 64% decrease.

Cocaine was administered on the third of the four FST days. As seen in Figure 2, a modest yet non-significant difference is seen between the adolescents and adults that received 5.0 mg/kg cocaine. A significant difference was seen between adolescents and adults at the 10.0 mg/kg, 20.0 mg/kg, and 40.0 mg/kg doses, with the adults spending more time immobile at each dose. The difference between adolescent and adults across the cocaine dose-response curve is further highlighted by examination of the difference data (i.e., cocaine data minus previous saline control day data). As noted with the FST: Cocaine Difference Values, Immobility Graph, the pattern of behavior noted in adolescence is dramatically different than that of adults with adolescents showing a systematic decrease in immobility across dose except at the highest dose. Predictably, when examining swimming data, a similar but reverse pattern of behavior is noted compared to immobility. Again, especially dramatic differences were noted with adolescent subjects showing robust swimming compared with adults as noted by examination of the raw and difference data (see, FST: Cocaine Test Values, Swimming Graph and Difference Values). Again, only a slight and non-significant difference is seen between the two groups at the 5.0 mg/kg dose. However, a significant difference is noted at the 10.0 mg/kg, 20.0 mg/kg, and 40.0 mg/kg doses; with the adolescents spending more time swimming. FST: Cocaine Test Values, Climbing Graph shows a significant difference at the 5.0 mg/kg dose, with the adolescents spending more time climbing than the adults. At the 10.0 mg/kg dose, the adults spend more time climbing, however, the difference was not significant. At the 20.0 mg/kg dose, the adolescents spend significantly more time climbing than the adults; and at the 40.0 mg/kg dose, the adolescents still spend more time climbing, but the difference is not significant.

As indicated in Figure 3 the change in immobility from the first saline day to the drug day at the 5.0 mg/kg dose is not significant when comparing the adolescent and adult groups. A significant difference is seen at both the 10.0 mg/kg and 20.0 mg/kg doses, with the adolescents having a decrease in immobility at both points. The difference seen at the 40.0 mg/kg dose is not significant. Similarly, difference data shows that the change in swimming from the first saline day to drug day is significant at all cocaine doses. The difference between the adults that received 5.0 mg/kg cocaine and the adults that received 10.0 mg/kg cocaine is significant; while the differences seen between adults that received 10.0 mg/kg and adults that received 20.0 mg/kg cocaine, as well as adults that received 20.0 mg/kg and adults that received the 40.0 mg/kg cocaine are not significant.

Considering the forced swim test is a method used in the measurement of despair, it is important to point out that the greatest overall response in the study was seen among the adolescents in immobility and, alternately, swimming. Previous studies have also reported a drastic response in adolescents to immobility, further supporting the importance of the forced swim test in showing the differences that exist between adolescents and adults (Bolanos et al., 2003). From childhood to adolescence, the instance of anxiety and depression increase significantly (Bolanos et al., 2003). Furthermore, adolescents are more susceptible to the impact of stress than adults are, and also show increased physiological responses when compared to those who are younger (Bolanos et al., 2003). While these finding are not entirely consistent with our study, our study did note a more dramatic response to cocaine, a drug abused for its mood lifting qualities.

It is susceptibility to and related lack of coping skills to stress and anxiety that often leads to drug abuse during adolescence (Bolanos et al., 2003). As a result of this vulnerability, teens may choose to use drugs as a means of self-medicating. Cocaine itself is more effective in the purpose of alleviating despair than in the purpose of achieving euphoria, in this study, which could be viewed as a worse-case scenario. If a teen is using cocaine as a way to feel less depressed, he or she will continue using the drug because cocaine makes him feel closer to normal or baseline behavior. The problem arises when tolerance develops, which happens rather quickly in adolescence, as noted by the motor activity data. Abusing cocaine for the euphoric effect may not produce the expected response, thus requiring higher doses to achieve and maintain an intoxicating state.

Activity testing also confirmed innate differences between adolescent and adults as noted by modest reductions in activity across saline test days. Additionally, the results from motor activity testing showed there was a statistically significant difference in the activity between the adolescents and adults across the cocaine dose-response curve. The difference between the adolescent and adult mice is magnified across the dose-response curve. For example, when 5 mg/kg of cocaine was administered, there is a significant difference in the levels of motor activity between the adolescents and the adults—with the adolescents displaying less activity. Though we found no statistically significant difference in the activity levels at the 10 mg/kg dose of cocaine, the adolescent subjects still show more rapid within session tolerance as noted by a steeper slope compared with the adults. In fact, across the entire dose-response curve, while cocaine caused an increase in activity at each dose, adolescents showed a more rapid decline in cocaine-induced motor activity within each session as noted by a stepper slope. As the dose increased, there was a rapid decline in the adolescents' motor activity; the slope for adolescent activity becomes much steeper when compared to the adults. The difference is most evident during testing with 20 mg/kg and 40 mg/kg cocaine, with the greatest changes in percentage of difference in activity and a much steeper slope for the adolescence. Across the entire cocaine dose-response curve at no point did adolescent show higher activity compared with adults; however, across most of the dose response curve adolescent subjects did show reduced activity compared with adults and this was further noted by a statistically significant change in slope compared to adults across every dose of cocaine. Taken together, this data provides convincing evidence that adolescent mice, compared with adults, are less sensitive to the motor activating effects of cocaine. This effect is consistent with previous reports (Kelley and Middaugh, 1999; Kelley and Rowan, 2004; Nolley and Kelley, 2007). Motor activating effects of psychostimulants are known to be correlated with their euphoric properties (Kelley and Berridge, 2002). This is noted in this study as well considering that motor activity was reduced in adolescent compared to adults across a cocaine dose-response curve and the same pattern was noted during CPP testing.

As shown in the Conditioned Place Preference graph (Figure 5), the adult subjects showed a greater all around response to change in preference than did the adolescents noting an increased sensitivity to the rewarding properties of cocaine.

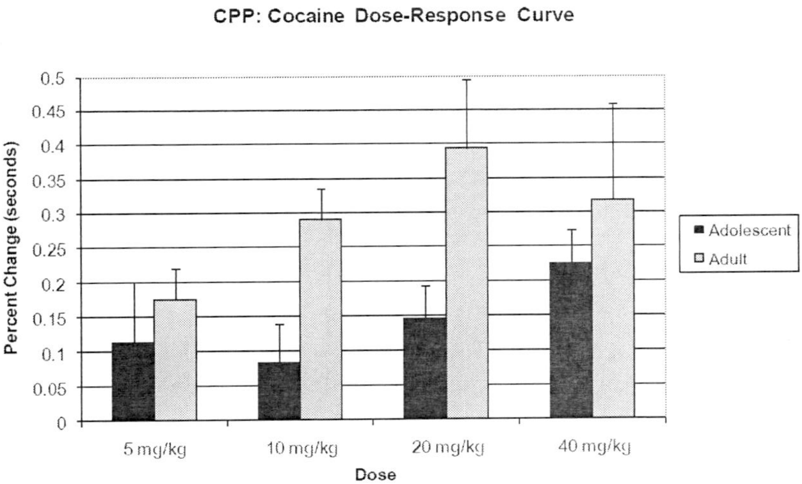

Figure 5. The effects of cocaine (5.0, 10.0, 20.0, and 40.0 mg/kg, IP injection) on conditioned-place-preference in adolescent and adult subjects (between subject design). Data is graphed as percent change in seconds (mean ± S.E.) on the non-preferred side of the condition-place-preference apparatus due to repeated cocaine pairings (post-test–pre-test/pre-test).

Although there were only moderate differences in percent change at the lowest and highest doses of 5 mg/kg and 40 mg/kg (i.e., with adults still showing a greater response compared to adolescents), there were significant differences in response at the 10 mg/kg and 20 mg/kg doses. This pattern was expected considering that the 5 mg/kg dose is considered a below threshold dose in this paradigm.

The highest dose of cocaine likely shows a drop in conditioning, from the previous dose, for the adults, because the adverse effects are beginning to distract from its rewarding effects. There is also a shift to the right of the dose response curve for the adolescents, an indication that the ceiling effect of cocaine for their population would presumably be reached at a higher dose. For the adolescents, the largest change in preference is seen at 40 mg/kg where in the adults the largest percent change in preference is shown at the 20 mg/kg dose. The differences at the 10 and 20 mg/kg doses exemplify the tendency for adolescents to switch preference based on reward factors which is a key piece of support toward the notion that human adolescents will seek novel and more potent drugs in order to satisfy the reward circuits of serotonin, dopamine, and norepinephrine. The decreased sensitivity in adolescent compared to adults was also noted with a less steep slope compared to adults indicating less of a change in reward across the dose-response curve.

Previous studies have also shown that the differences between adolescents and adults in response to reward are exemplified by the conditioned place preference test. These differences are enhanced when a precursor of several days of MDMA (Ecstasy) injections are given prior to the cocaine conditioned place preference (Abreu-Villaca et al., 2003). The adults receiving both the MDMA and the cocaine showed a higher preference for the side paired with drug, while the adolescents receiving the same treatment did not significantly change preference. Similar findings were noted with cocaine and methylphenidate indicating, again, that adolescent subjects require a greater dose of a rewarding drug to fully appreciate its rewarding effects. Behaviorally, this could be seen as consuming more drugs to achieve euphoria or consuming the drug faster or even a combination of the two. Either way, increase drug dose increases risk for abuse, dependence, and adverse events.

Decreased sensitivity to a drug is likely to lead to abuse and dependence, especially in adolescence due to the need for increased amount and/or frequency of administration (Schuckit, 1993, 1994). The drug also serves not only as a positive reinforcer to elevate mood from despair to normal, as noted in CPP, but also as a negative reinforcer to elevate depressed mood back to normal or euphoria, as noted in FST. It has already been shown that early exposure to nicotine leads to more frequent exposures and the increased likelihood of depression, which in turn increases the chances of adolescents using nicotine again as a negative reinforcer (Achat-Mendes, Anderson, and Itzhak, 2003). Unfortunately, adolescence is an opportune time to engage in drug use because of the adolescents' belief that drugs will elevate depressed mood (Anderson, 2003; Chen and Miller, 1998) and this is the time period during which the drug is most likely to result in abuse and dependence. For this reason, addiction is largely considered to be a pediatric phenomenon where adolescent drug use carries over into adulthood.

Since adolescents have affective states and responses to pharmacological stimuli that are different than adults, lasting changes due to acute or chronic substance exposure during adolescence, such as desensitization, may indicate permanent alterations in neural function. Extending the concept of a longitudinal deviation in developmental trajectory, drug use during adolescents may cause not only aberrant maturation but may abrogate certain aspects of neurodevelopment thereby causing a perseveration of the adolescent condition or worsening of any psychopathology. For those adolescents at risk for various psychological disorders, the use of abused substances during this critical period of development may increase, in intensity and frequency, the exact psychological state they are trying to alter, thus, perpetuating a cycle in which greater use of an abused drug, in intensity and frequency, will be required to achieve a desired immediate effect but giving rise to greater psychopathology across time. Given the nature of this cycle and its impact on brain development, such a pattern of use may result in permanent changes in important neurobiological systems resulting in even greater risk for continued, perhaps permanent, substance abuse and affective disorders.

While cocaine was selected for testing in this study, nearly all abused drugs seem to work, in part, through activation of the dopaminergic system. For example, an in vivo microdialysis study demonstrated that nicotine as well as amphetamine, ethanol, cocaine and opiates increased extracellular dopamine in the nucleus accumbens of freely moving rats (Di Chiara and Imperato, 1988). In contrast, drugs with aversive properties reduced extracelluar dopamine in this region, while drugs not abused by humans failed to have any effect on extracellular dopamine (Di Chiara and Imperato, 1988). The dopaminergic systems within the nucleus accumbens is also involved with the locomotor effects of many abused drugs. For example, the locomotor activating properties of the psychomotor stimulants, the opiates, caffeine, barbiturates, alcohol, benzodiazapines, cannabis, and phencyclidine appear to be neuronally linked to their reinforcing effects (Wise and Bozarth, 1987). Therefore, it is likely, even probable, that other abused drugs will produce similar results. However, further testing will be required to elucidate this developmental phenomenon.

Although this study addresses several important effects of cocaine on adolescent behavior compared to adults, further studies on this topic are required to more fully explain the effect of adolescent drug exposure. While our study provided original and important finding with important implications for human behavior, our study included several important limitations. For example, our study did not examine these differences in respect to female subjects, which would be valuable especially in regards to despair because of the prevalence of depression among the female population is twice that of males (Adriani and Laviola, 2004). There have been previous studies that utilized the same testing procedures using male rats and similar results were found (Abreu-Villaca et al., 2003). However, it is necessary to conduct similar studies on several animal species and strains in order to have full support and documentation of the concluding results. Even within the same strain of species, young adolescents may differ from older adolescents because of the transitional nature of the critical period (Bresula and Peterson, 1996). It is therefore imperative that our results be repeated across species and within species strains. Furthermore, it is possible that adolescents show an initial period of increased sensitivity to abused drugs followed by rapid tolerance; however, our study was not able to examine this possibility. Because there can be differing interpretations of data and results, full examination of the relationship between adolescents and cocaine in regards to despair is desirable. It would be valuable to determine the tolerance rate of adolescents when they are regularly being exposed to cocaine doses. In conclusion, the implications of this study are clinically relevant and could help provide new avenues for prevention and treatment strategies for our youth. For example, according to this study, adolescents have reduced sensitivity to the rewarding effects of cocaine and, as such, an appropriate adaptive response to reduced sensitivity is to administer higher amounts and at greater frequencies. On the other hand, if cocaine is especially effective as a negative reinforcer in adolescents, for a common psychological problem, its potential for abuse would be profoundly elevated in this age group compared to any other. Combined, these findings suggest possible course for substance abuse in adolescents and a subsequent cycle of abuse. Related, this finding is of particular relevance in terms of a neurobiological "gateway drug effects," and may generalize to other drugs of abuse like alcohol, amphetamines, or opioids.

Acknowledgments

This research was supported by the Thomas F. Jeffress and Kate Miller Jeffress Memorial Trust and by Bridgewater College. We thank Laura Low, Ashley Furr, Sherri Ferland, Cammy Huston, and Todd Mitchem for their help with this project.

References

Aberg M., D. Wade, E. Wall, S. Izenwasser, Effect of MDMA (ecstasy) on activity and cocaine conditioned place preference in adult and adolescent rats, *Neurotoxicol teratol 29* (2007) 37-46.

Abreu-Villaca Y., F.J. Seidler, C.A. Tate, T.A. Slotkin, Nicotine is a neurotoxin in the adolescent brain: critical periods, patterns of exposure, regional selectivity, and dose thresholds for macromolecular alterations, *Brain Res.* 979 (2003) 114-128.

Achat-Mendes C., K.L. Anderson, Y. Itzhak, Methylphenidate and MDMA adolescent exposure in mice; long-lasting consequences on cocaine-induced reward and psychomotor stimulation in adulthood, *Neuropharmacology* 45 (2003) 106-115.

Adriani W., G. Laciola, Windows of vulnerability to psychopathology and therapeutic strategy in the adolescent rodent model, *Behav. Pharmacol.* 15 (2004) 341-352.

Altman J., S.A. Bayer, Migration and distribution of two populations of hippocampal granule cell precursors during the perinatal and postnatal periods, *J. Comp. Neurol.* 301 (1990) 365-381.

Anderson S.L., Trajectories of brain development point of vulnerability or window of opportunity? *Neurosci. Biobehav. Rev.* 27 (2003) 3-18.

Anderson S.L., Stimulants and the developing brain, *Trends Pharmacol. Sci.* 26 (2005) 237-253.

Bayer S.A., J.W. Yackel, P.S. Puri, Neurons in the rate dentate gyrus granular layer substantially increase during juvenile and adult life, *Science* 216 (1982) 890–892.

Bolanos C.A., M.B. Barrot, O. Berton, D. Wallace-Black, E.J. Nestler, Methylphenidate treatment during pre- and periadolescence alters behavioral responses to emotional stimuli at adulthood, *Biol. Psychiatry* 54 (2003) 1317–1329.

Bresula N., E.L. Peterson, Smoking cessation in young adults: age at initiation of cigarette smoking and other suspected influences, *Am. J. Publ. Health* 86 (1996) 214–220.

Burke KC, Burke JD, Regier DA, Rae DS. Age at onset of selected mental disorders in five community populations. *Arch Gen Psychiatry* 1990;47:511–518. [PubMed: 2350203].

Carelzon W.A. Jr., S.D. Mague, S.L. Anderson, Enduring behavioral effects of early exposure to methylphenidate in rats, *Biol. Psychiatry* 54 (2003) 1330–1337.

Chambers R.A., J.R. Taylor, M.N. Potenza, Developmental neurocircuitry of motivation in adolescence: a critical period of addiction vulnerability, *Am. J. Psychiatry* 160 (2003) 1041–1052.

Chen K, Kandel DB, Davies M. Relationships between frequency and quantity of marijuana use and last year proxy dependence among adolescents and adults in the United States. *Drug Alcohol Depend* 1997;46:53–67. [PubMed: 9246553].

Chen J., W.J. Millar, Age of smoking initiation: implications for quitting, *Health Rep.* 9 (1998) 39–46.

Clark DB, Kirisci L, Tarter RE. Adolescent versus adult onset and the development of substance use disorders in males. *Drug Alcohol Depend* 1998;49:115–21. [PubMed: 9543648]

Cryan JF, Markou A, Lucki I. Assessing antidepressant activity in rodents: recent developments and future needs. *Trends Pharmacol Sci* 2002;23:238–246. [PubMed: 12008002].

De La Garza R., J.J. Mahoney III, A distinct neurochemical profile in WKY rats at baseline and in response to acute stress: implications for animal models of anxiety and depression, *Brain Res.* 1021(2004) 209-218.

Detke MJ, Rickels M, Lucki I. Active behaviors in the rat forced swimming test differentially produced by serotonergic and noradrenergic antidepressants. *Psychopharmacology* 1995;121:66–72. [PubMed: 8539342].

Estroff TW, Schwartz RH, Hoffmann NG. Adolescent cocaine abuse — addictive potential, behavioraland psychiatric effects. *Clin Pediatr* 1989;28:550–5.

Giaconia RM, Reinherz HZ, Silverman AB, Pakiz B, Frost AK, Cohen E. Ages of onset of psychiatric disorders in a community population of older adolescents. *J Am Acad Child Adolesc Psychiatry* 1994;33:706–717. [PubMed: 8056734].

Ginzel K. H., G. S. Maritz, D. F. Marks, M. Neuberger, J. R. Pauly, J. R. Polito, R. Schulte-Hermann, T. A. Slotkin, Critical Review: Nicotine for the Fetus, the Infant and the Adolescent?, *J. Health Psych* 12 (2007) 215-224.

Hankin BL, Abramson LY, Moffitt TE, Silva PA, McGee R, Angell KE. Development of depression from preadolescence to young adulthood: emerging gender differences in a 10-year longitudinal study. *J Abnorm Psychol* 1998;107:128–140. [PubMed: 9505045]

Hildebrandt M. G., K. B. Stage, P. Kragh-Soerensen, Gender and depression: a study of severity and symptomatology of depressive disorders (ICD-10) in general practice, *Acta Psychiatrica Scandinavica* 107 (2003) 197-202.

Hohn KG, Wuttke W. Ontogeny of catecholamine turnover rates in limbic and hypothalamic structures in relation to serum prolactin and gonadotropin levels. *Brain Res* 1979;179:281–293. [PubMed:574418]

Huttenlocher P.R., Morphometric study of human cerebral cortex development, *Neuropsychologia* 29 (1990) 517–527.

Izenwasser S., Differential Effects Of Psychoactive Drugs In Adolescents and Adults, *Crit Rev Neurobiol* 17 (2005) 51-67.

Kalsbeek A, Voorn P, Buijs RM, Pool CW, Uylings HB. Development of the dopaminergic innervations in the prefrontal cortex of the rat. *J Comp Neurol* 1988;269:58–72. [PubMed: 3361004]

Kelley A.E and Berridge K.C. The neuroscience of natural rewards: relevance to addictive drugs. *J. Neurosci*. 2002 May 1;22(9):3303-5.

Kelley, B.M., Middaugh, L.D., 1999b. Periadolescent nicotine exposure reduces cocaine reward in adult mice. *J. Addict*. Dis. 18, 27–39.

Kelley B.M., J.D. Rowan, Long-term, low-level adolescent nicotine exposure produces dose-development changes in cocaine sensitivity and reward in adult mice, *Int J Devl Neurosci* 22 (2004) 339-348.

Klimek V., J.E. Schenck, H. Han, C.A. Stockmeier, G.A. Ordway, Dopaminergic abnormalities in amygdaloid nuclei in major depression: a postmodern study, *Biol. Psychiatry* 52 (2002) 740-748.

Koe B.K., Molecular geometry of inhibitors of the uptake of catecholamines and serotonin in synaptosomal preparations of rat brain, *J Pharmacol Exp Ther* 199 (1976) 649–661.

Lewinsohn PM, Clarke GN, Seely JR, Rohde P. Major depression in community adolescents: age at onset, episode duration and time to recurrence. *J Am Acad Child Adolesc Psych* 1994;140:809–818.

Lidow MS, Goldman-Rakic PS, Rakic P. Synchronized overproduction of neurotransmitter receptors in diverse regions of the primate cerebral cortex. *Proc Natl Acad Sci U S A* 1991;88:10218–10221. [PubMed: 1658799]

Little K.Y., D.M. Krolewski, L. Zhang, B.J. Cassin, Loss of striatal vesicular monoamine transporter protein (VMAT2) in human cocaine users, Am. *J. Psychiatry* 160 (2003) 45-47.

McWilliams J.R., G. Lynch, Rate of synaptic replacement in degenerate rate hippocampus declines precipitously from the juvenile period to adulthood, *Science* 221 (1983) 572–574.

The National Center on Addiction and Substance Abuse at Columbia University (CASA), Tobbacco : *The Smoking Gun* (2007).

[NIDA] National Institute of Drug Abuse. Drug Abuse and Addiction: One of America's Most Challenging Public Health Problems. *<http://www.nida.nih.gov/about/welcome/aboutdrugabuse/magnitude/>* Accessed 2008, Mar 8.

Nolley E.P., B.M. Kelley, Adolescent reward system perseveration due to nicotine: Studies with methylphenidate, *Neurotoxicol Teratol* 29 (2007) 47-56.

Porsolt RD, Le Pichon M, Jalfre M. Depression: a new animal model sensitive to antidepressant treatments. *Nature* 1997;266:730–732. [PubMed: 559941]

Reith M.E., M.Y. Li, Q.S. Yan, Extracellular dopamine, norepinephrine, and serotonin in the ventral tegmental area and nucleus accumbens of freely moving rats during intracerebral dialysis following systemic administration of cocaine and other uptake blockers. *Psychopharmacology* 134 (1997) 309–317.

Rezvani A.H., E.D. Levin, Adolescent and adult rats respond differently to nicotine and alcohol: motor activity and body temperature, *Int. J. Dev. Neurosci.* 22 (2004) 349–354.

Robins LN, Przybeck TR. Age of onset of drug use as a factor in drug and other disorders. *NIDA Res Monogr* 1995;56:178–92. [PubMed: 3929100]

Rocha B.A., E.H. Goulding, L.E. O'Dell, A.N. Mead, N.G. Coufal, L.H. Parsons, L.H. Tecott, Enhanced Locomotor, Reinforcing, and Neurochemical Effects of Cocaine in Serotonin 5-Hydroxytryptamine 2C Receptor Mutant Mice, *J. Neurosci* 22 (2002) 10039-10045.

Salamone J.D., M. Correa, S. Mingote, S.M. Weber, Nucleus accumbens dopamine and the regulation of effort in food-seeking behavior: implications for studies of natural motivation, psychiatry, and drug abuse, *J. Pharmacol. Exp. Ther*. 305 (2003) 1-8.

[SAMSHA] Substance Abuse and Mental Health Services Administration. 2007, Oct 12. Results from the 2006 National Survey on Drug Use and Health: National Findings.<*http://oas.samhsa.gov/nsduh/2k6nsduh/ 2k6Results.cfm#2.2*> Accessed 2008, Mar 8.

Scheetz A.J., M. Constantine-Paton, Modulation of NMDA receptor function: implications for vertebrate neural development, *FASEB J.* 8 (1994) 745–752.

Schuckit, M.A., 1993. Reaction to alcohol as a predictor of alcoholism. *Alcohol Alcohol.* 2, 91–91.

Schuckit, M.A., 1994. Low level of response to alcohol as a predictor of future alcoholism. *Am. J. Psychiatry* 151, 184–189.

Shalaby IA, Dendel PS, Spear LP. Differential functional ontogeny of dopamine presynaptic receptor regulation. *Brain Res* 1981;227:434–439. [PubMed: 7260651]

Slotkin T.A., Cholinergic systems in brain development and disruption by neurotoxicants: nicotine, environmental tobacco smoke, *organophosphates, Toxicol. Appl. Pharmacol.* 198 (2004) 132–151.

Spear L.P., S.C. Brake, Periadolescence: age-dependent behavior and psychopharmacological responsivity in rats, *Dev. Psychobiol.* 16 (1983) 83–109.

Spear L.P., The adolescent brain and age-related behavioral manifestations, *Neurosci Behav Rev* 24 (2000) 417-463.

Spear L., Modeling adolescent development and alcohol use in animals, *Alcohol Research and Health* 24 (2000) 115-123.

Spear L. P., Adolescent Brain Development and Animal Models, *Ann. N.Y. Acad. Sci.* 1021 (2004) 23-26.

Teicher MH, Andersen SL, Hostetter JC Jr. Evidence for dopamine receptor pruning between adolescence and adulthood in striatum but not nucleus accumbens. *Dev Brain Res* 1995;89:167–172. [PubMed: 8612321]

Teslik L.H., Council on Foreign Relations. 2006, April 6. The Forgotten Drug War. <*http://www.cfr.org/publication/10373/#3*> Accessed 2008, Mar 8.

Torabi M.R., W.J. Bailey, M. Majd-Jabbari, Cigarette smoking as a predictor of alcohol and other drug use by children and adolescents: evidence of the "gateway drug effect", *J Sch Health* 63 (1993) 302-306.

Valentino R. J., J. F. Cryan, I. Lucki, Assessing Substrates underlying the behavioral effects of antidepressants using the modified rat forced swimming test, *Neurosci and Behav. Reviews* 29 (2005) 547-569.

Vidrine J. I., C. B. Anderson, K. I. Pollack, D. W. Wetter, Gender Differences in Adolescent smoking: mediator and moderator effects of self-generated expected smoking outcomes, *American Journal of Health Promotion* 20 (2006) 383-387.

Weissman MM, Warner V, Wickramaratne P, Moreau D, Olfson M. Offspring of depressed parents. 10 years later. *Arch Gen Psychiatry* 1997;54:932–940. [PubMed: 9337774]

Willner P. Animal models of depression: an overview. *Pharmac Ther* 1990;45:425–455.

Wise, R.A. Neural mechanism of the reinforcing action of cocaine. *NIDA Res Monogr* 50 (1984) 15.

Wood, W.G. H.J. Armbrecht, R.W. Wise, Ethanol intoxication and withdrawal among three age groups of C57BL/6NNIA mice, *Pharmacol Biochem Behav* (1982) 17 1037-1041.

Index

Index

M

N

O

P

R

S